Gluten F[ree]

Go Gluten Free Now! How And Why You Should Avoid Gluten

By Steve Rowland

© Copyright 2015 by Steve Rowland - All rights reserved.

This document is geared towards providing exact and reliable information in regards to the topic and issue covered. The publication is sold with the idea that the publisher is not required to render accounting, officially permitted, or otherwise, qualified services. If advice is necessary, legal or professional, a practiced individual in the profession should be ordered.

- From a Declaration of Principles which was accepted and approved equally by a Committee of the American Bar Association and a Committee of Publishers and Associations.

In no way is it legal to reproduce, duplicate, or transmit any part of this document in either electronic means or in printed format. Recording of this publication is strictly prohibited and any storage of this document is not allowed unless with written permission from the publisher. All rights reserved.

The information provided herein is stated to be truthful and consistent, in that any liability, in terms of inattention or otherwise, by any usage or abuse of any policies, processes, or directions contained within is the solitary and utter responsibility of the recipient reader. Under no circumstances will any legal responsibility or blame be held against the publisher for any reparation, damages, or monetary loss due to the information herein, either directly or indirectly.

Respective authors own all copyrights not held by the publisher.

The information herein is offered for informational purposes solely, and is universal as so. The presentation of the information is without contract or any type of guarantee assurance.

The trademarks that are used are without any consent, and the publication of the trademark is without permission or backing by the trademark owner. All trademarks and brands within this book are for clarifying purposes only and are the owned by the owners themselves, not affiliated with this document.

Disclaimer – Please read!

The information provided in this book is designed to provide helpful information on the subjects discussed. This book is not meant to be used, nor should it be used, to diagnose or treat any medical condition. For diagnosis or treatment of any medical problem, consult your own physician. The publisher and author are not responsible for any specific health or allergy needs that may require medical supervision and are not liable for any damages or negative consequences from any treatment, action, application or preparation, to any person reading or following the information in this book. References are provided for informational purposes only and do not constitute endorsement of any websites or other sources. Readers should be aware that the websites listed in this book may change.

Table Of Contents

Introduction 9
Chapter One - What exactly is Gluten, and Which Foods Contain It? 11
What is Gluten? 11
What Foods Contain Gluten? 11
How Widespread is Gluten in the Average Person's Diet? 13
Avoiding High-Gluten Foods 13
What Food Groups to Delete from Your Diet 14
Chapter Two – Just How Detrimental Is Gluten to Health? 19
Gluten and the Immune System 20
Gluten Affects Disease Development 21
Brain Disorders and Gluten 21
Non-Celiac Gluten Sensitivity Studies 24
Other Predictive Health Issue Examples 28
Gluten Effects on the Brain 29
When Are Full Benefits Achieved after Going Gluten-Free? .. 30
The Gluten Free Summit 32
Gluten's Effects on the Intestine 34
Gluten and Fibromyalgia 36
Why Some Physicians Recommend Going Gluten-Free 37
Chapter Three - How to Make the Transition to Gluten-Free Foods – and Avoid the Common Mistakes! 41
Chapter Four – Great, Healthy Gluten-Free Diet Planning 53
What Can You Eat? 53
Baking without Gluten 54
The Cost of Going Gluten-Free 56
What to Look for on Food Packaging 58
10 Delicious Gluten Free Breakfast Recipes 67
GLUTEN FREE PANCAKES 67

6

SCRAMBLED TOFU 69
CINNAMON QUINOA PORRIDGE.. 70
BAKED EGGS IN A PORTOBELLO MUSHROOM.................. 71
VERY BERRY OMLETTE 72
BAKED FRUITS WITH VANILLA..73
SPICY TOMATO BAKED EGGS 74
ORANGE POLENTA 75
CRISPY POTATOES WITH GREEN BEANS AND EGGS........76
CREAMY BANANA BUCKWHEAT PORRIDGE......................77

10 Delicious Gluten Free Lunch Recipes 79
SPICY TUNA POTATO 79
CHICKEN CAESAR SALAD... 80
POTATO, LEEK AND PARMESAN FRITATTA 81
BUCKWHEAT NOODLE SALAD WITH CHICKEN AND
SCALLIONS 83
SPICY BUTTERNUT AND APPLE SOUP.............................. 84
MINTY CARROT AND FETA SALAD 85
SPICED QUINOA WITH ALMONDS AND FETA................. 86
SWEET POTATO WITH RICOTTA AND KALE 87
AVOCADO WITH A BLACK BEAN SALSA.......................... 88
RICE NOODLES WITH A BROCCOLI AND ALMOND PESTO
.... 89

10 Delicious Gluten Free Dinner Recipes................. 91
ORANGE AND HONEY SEA BASS WITH LENTILS 91
SHERRY CHICKEN WITH ALMONDS AND DATES 93
ROSEMARY CHICKEN WITH A TOMATO SAUCE.............95
GLUTEN FREE MACARONI CHEESE 96
CHICKEN AND LEEK PIE 98
GLUTEN FREE PIZZA DOUGH.. 100
MEATBALL AND BUTTERBEAN STEW 101
MISO ROASTED AUBERGINE STEAKS WITH SWEET
POTATO 102
WARM QUINOA SALAD WITH HALLOUMI 103
ROSEMARY LAMB CHOPS WITH ROASTED POTATOES.104

7

10 Delicious Gluten Free Dessert Recipes 105
CHOCOLATE POTS 105
POACHED PEARS... 106
MAPLE AND WALNUT BAKED APPLES 107
PEACH AND RASPBERRY PARFAIT................................ 108
RASPBERRY FOOL.. 109
EASY CHOCOLATE RICOTTA MOUSSE 110
CARAMELIZED PINEAPPLE WITH A COCONUT SORBERT
.... 111
BUTTERMILK PUDDING 112
RASPBERRY SORBET WITH MERINGUES 113
MANGO GRATIN 114

10 Delicious Gluten Free Side Dish/Appetizer Recipes 115
SPINACH AND ARTICHOKE DIP 115
CRISPY BAKED KALE CHIPS 116
HAM ROLL UPS..117
ASPARAGUS WRAPPED IN PROSCIUTTO 118
BACON AND DATES APPETIZERS 119
STUFFED CELERY 120
BEETROOT HUMMUS 121
ROASTED SWEET ONION DIP 122
ROSEMARY, FENNEL AND CITRUS OLIVES 123
HONEY ROASTED FRUIT AND NUTS............................ 124

Conclusion 125
Free Ebook Offer...127

8

Introduction

For years, it has been known that gluten causes damage for people with celiac disease. What was not widely known until recently is that gluten also has damaging effects on people who are not affected with celiac disease. Early research has suggested that gluten sensitivity among non-celiacs is a natural reaction of the human immune system.

Gluten should be avoided not only by those who have Celiac disease, but by the general public, as well. The only difference between these people is the stronger reaction of those with Celiac disease to gluten and wheat. Even people who have no indications of the disease have some type of reaction to the consumption of Gluten.

Gluten causes inflammation of the gut in 80% or more of the population. That's a huge percentage of people who can benefit from a gluten-free diet. Most people develop antibodies in the gut, against gluten proteins. What this means is that every time you consume gluten, your body is having an immune system reaction to it. This is what causes a lot of the health problems for many people. It simply isn't healthy for the body to be having a reaction every single time you consume gluten, which for most people is every meal! 99% of people have the potential, genetically, to develop antibodies against gluten. Yet nobody has the ability to fully digest Gluten.

Antibodies that act in the stomach, surprisingly, can be a good thing. When your body does not react against the intrusion of gluten immediately, the gluten proteins might more easily enter the bloodstream. This would trigger immune reactions in other parts of the body.

The main gluten protein that causes problems is Gliadin. It is structurally similar to other proteins found in the Pancreas and Thyroid. Antibodies that fight Gliadin might also attack these organs themselves, causing autoimmune problems like type 1 diabetes and hypothyroidism.

Humans are not adapted to properly eat and digest wheat. Sadly, wheat is ever-present in our foods and our society. Many health conditions might not even exist if wheat was not as highly consumed.

You will notice positive changes almost immediately after you remove wheat and other grains that contain gluten from your diet. This book will lead you through the process of eliminating gluten from your diet, and giving you viable alternatives that can satisfy hunger without the dangers of gluten. Your body will thank you for adopting a gluten-free diet.

Chapter One - What exactly is Gluten, and Which Foods Contain It?

What is Gluten?

Gluten is in its simplest form a name for the proteins that one finds in wheat, barley, rye and triticale. Wheat includes einkorn, khorasan wheat, faro, farina, spelt, emmer and durum. Gluten is used to help foods in maintaining their shape. It effectively holds foods together. Some foods you would never think of as containing gluten actually do. The main three gluten-filled foods are wheat, rye and barley.

What Foods Contain Gluten?

In addition to wheat, rye and barley, foods that contain malt have gluten. They include malt vinegar, malt flavoring, malt syrup, malt extract, malted milk, malted milkshakes and malted barley flour. Brewer's yeast is also a culprit.

Many foods that contain gluten sources may have the ingredient hidden within the list of ingredients. Be sure to read labels before you assume that a product is gluten-free. Some products labeled wheat-free are actually not gluten-free. They could still contain rye, barley or spelt, which is contain gluten.

Common foods with gluten among their ingredients are:

- Beer (unless it is listed as explicitly gluten-free)
- Malt beverages
- Noodles, including egg noodles, chow mein and ramen. Mung bean and rice noodles are free of gluten.
- Pastas, including gnocchi, couscous, dumplings and ravioli
- Pastries and breads, including rolls, doughnuts, muffins, potato bread, cornbread, flatbreads, bagels, pita and croissants
- Brownies, pie crusts, cookies and cakes
- Crackers, including graham crackers, Goldfish® and pretzels
- Cereals like rice puffs and corn flakes made with malt flavoring or extract
- Granola, if made with regular, not gluten-free, oats
- Flour tortillas
- Breakfast foods, like biscuits, crepes, French toast, waffles and pancakes
- Coating and breading mixes
- Gravies and sauces, if they use wheat flour to thicken the product, as well as cream sauces and soy sauce
- Croutons, dressings and stuffing

- Any other food that includes "wheat flour"
- It is important to point out that this not an exhaustive list and that it is absolutely essential you thoroughly check a products ingredients list.

How Widespread is Gluten in the Average Person's Diet?

The average person's daily diet contains between 10 and 40 grams of gluten. This includes gluten found in whole wheat bread and pasta.

Avoiding High-Gluten Foods
Gluten causes problems for people with Celiac disease, as well as for people who have a milder intolerance for gluten. Gluten intolerance has the potential to lead to Chrohn's disease and rheumatoid arthritis. It can cause other symptoms, including headaches, skin rashes and irritable bowel syndrome. Avoiding foods that contain gluten will help alleviate most symptoms.

Giving up gluten is not easy. Wheat is the flour most often used for commercial cereals, baked goods and pastas. Staying away from it may seem overwhelming and challenging, at first. There are many gluten-free products available today, as bakeries and food manufacturers respond to the increase in demand. Another important idea here – Gluten free junk food is still junk food. For example a gluten free chocolate muffin is still unhealthy, plenty of people assume the gluten free label means the product must be healthy. This is not true!

What Food Groups to Delete from Your Diet

Grains

You must avoid some grains, so that you do not experience gluten reactions. This includes all of these foods:

Bread, pasta, muffins, cereals, cookies, bagels, gravies, cakes, bread crumbs, croutons, rolls, biscuits, pita bread, noodles, batter-fried foods, ice cream cones, wheat tortillas, wheat germ, bran, pancake mixes, dumplings, pies, pancake mixes, rye and pumpernickel bread, vermicelli, cornbread, buns, doughnuts, spaghetti, pretzels, pastries and waffles.

You can eat these products if they are labeled as gluten-free. Many grocery stores carry gluten-free versions of the foods above. You should leave many of these foods out of a diet simply because they are junk food.

Processed Meats

Physicians who deal with patients who have Celiac disease recommend eliminating processed meats from your diet, even if you are not highly symptomatic. Processed meats to avoid include pate, salami, pepperoni, bologna, sausages, hot dogs, liverwurst and cold cuts. Various grains with gluten may be used when they are made.

Alcoholic Beverages

A good gluten-free diet will include the elimination of alcoholic drinks, like light beer, ale and beer. You should also avoid hard liquors that are made with grains containing gluten. If you have been diagnosed with intolerance to gluten, you should proceed with caution to determine the level of your tolerance for alcoholic drinks. These include whiskey, some vodkas and most gin. There is a plethora of further benefits to cutting toxic Alcohol from your diet, but there is plenty of information out there regarding that.

Seasonings and Condiments

Many seasonings and condiments do contain gluten and can cause issues for you if you are intolerant to gluten. Unless the labels say gluten-free, eliminate MSG, Worcestershire sauce, soy sauce, barley malt, bouillon, malt products, modified food starch and any gravy or salad dressings that are thickened with flour that is wheat or otherwise gluten-based.

Sweets

This may be one of the hardest categories from which to stay away. Many treats include flour and other gluten sources. The sweets to avoid include malt products, chocolate candy that contains malt, candies with malt extract, ice cream, root beer, sherbets and commercial cake products. Check your labels carefully to ensure that you are choosing gluten-free foods.

Don't get too upset!

I remember when I was first researching which products contain gluten. I was so upset about all the foods that I thought were so great at the time. My disappointed was short lived you'll be glad to hear. The gluten free industry is exploding at the moment, tons of new businesses are creating really innovative and delicious products for us. Supermarket gluten free sections are growing and every day we are seeing more and more options to diversify our gluten free diets.

Cross Contamination

Even if you choose only gluten-free foods for your healthy diet, what if they are made in factories that also make products that contain gluten? Cross-contamination can also occur in your kitchen, when you are preparing meals for yourself and others. If you can use separate cutting boards and cooking utensils, this will help you from inadvertently adding gluten to your otherwise-healthy, gluten-free diet.

Chapter Two – Just How Detrimental Is Gluten to Health?

There are nearly 20,000 medical literature articles about sensitivity to gluten and how this affects your body. Thousands of research teams have looked at these issues and determined that they are indeed problems even for people without celiac disease.

Researchers feel that the problems caused by gluten may extend to juvenile idiopathic arthritis, Parkinson's and Alzheimer's. They have also touched on a connection between gluten and liver cancer and intestinal permeability.

Not only are researchers linking gluten to health issues, but more family and general practitioners are finding that between three and six people out of every 10 who visit with medical issues have elevated antibodies due to a gluten reaction. This means that the immune systems of these patients are telling physicians that there is, indeed, a problem.

There is no vast amount of money in conducting research on gluten sensitivity. No one is looking for a wonder drug that will profit companies. They are just discovering that the links between gluten and many body symptoms are real.

Gluten and the Immune System

Just because a food does not contain gluten doesn't mean that it is not junk food. Working with a dietician or nutritionist will be helpful in setting up a healthy diet that is also gluten-free.

Many general practitioners are not trained in the links between gluten and physical issues. When your immune system reacts to gluten, it works in much the same way as a vaccine. The body recognizes that gluten is not good for it, and takes steps to counter the effects.

The active part of the immune system is the memory-B cell. It does not go away. If your body reacts negatively to gluten, this means that your body has memory-B cells related to gluten. Any gluten can cause reactions, even small amounts. The antibodies can work for months after your body reacts to gluten. That is why is essential to cut gluten out fully, even one small bit after a month of being free can set of the body's reaction system all over again.

The human digestive system cannot digest gluten. The proteins found in wheat, rye and barley are not digestible by the human body. They are not broken down into dipeptides or triteptides like most foods are.

Gluten Affects Disease Development

If your body has gluteomorphins in the bloodstream, they affect the brain receptors that stimulate feel-good hormones. Eating too much gluten in your diet deregulates your receptors, and they no longer work.

This mechanism develops into type 2 diabetes. From your early life, you probably eat a lot of sugar, which deregulates the receptors for insulin, and they work less efficiently.

Similar effects are found when the peptides from poorly digested gluten hit your opiate receptors. The opiate receptors in your brain are downgraded. This is associated with anxiety, depression, autism and attention deficit disorder. This is also a reason why the main cognitive complaint with celiac disease is depression.

Brain Disorders and Gluten

Many brain disorders have a link to gluten, and patients often see dramatic improvement if they go on a gluten-free diet. Even though gluten primarily affects the gut, it can affect the brain as well. Neurological illnesses may be brought about or exacerbated by the intake of gluten. This field is known as gluten sensitive idiopathic neuropathy (GSIN).

In a study following patients with neurological illnesses of unknown causes, more than half of the 53 patients had antibodies in the blood against gluten. This is according to a 1996 study: Does cryptic gluten sensitivity play a part in neurological illness? As reported in the National Institutes of Health.

Gluten is believed to be at least partially to blame for cerebellar ataxia, in which patients cannot coordinate speech, movements and balance. Many ataxia cases are linked directly to the consumption of gluten. It leads to irreversible damage in the cerebellum.

Studies have shown associations, at least statistically, between the consumption of gluten and cerebellar ataxia. These patients often improve on gluten-free diets.
Schizophrenia and epilepsy patients sometimes see impressive improvements when they remove gluten from their diet.

Extensive Research in Finland About Underachievement Links to Gluten

Researchers in Finland have an ongoing study that ties in with cardiovascular disease. This is the top cause of death in Finland. They sent letters to 5000 adults with families, asking if they might follow the children to identify what mechanisms make them more vulnerable to the development of cardiovascular disease.

That research started 20 years ago. Nearly 2,500 young adults are still in this study. They kept in touch and were tested every year. Gathering information, researchers searched for patterns for any of these younger adults who might develop cardiovascular disease.

Other researchers used the blood drawn from these study patients and discovered that many had silent celiac disease. If they haven't yet experienced stomach symptoms, they don't know how the gluten is affecting them.

As it turned out, 50 of the nearly 2,500 people in the study had silent celiac. This means that the immune system was active with antibodies for gluten. Patients who were diagnosed with Celiac had half the number of people attending collage than those without Celiac.

In addition, patients in this study who have silent celiac are only promoted in their job about 20% of the time. Those who did not have silent celiac were promoted at a rate close to 50%.

This study was titled "Silent Celiac Disease: A Cause of Underachievement." Those who did not go on to higher education and promotions don't necessarily feel dissatisfied with their lives. But how much more could they have done if they hadn't been suffering the silent symptoms of celiac disease?

These 50 people had silent celiac. How many more people had gluten sensitivity that was not serious enough to be considered celiac disease? One more recent study shows that sensitivity to gluten is over 30 times as common as celiac disease itself.

Non-Celiac Gluten Sensitivity Studies

These studies just began several years ago. Researchers finally recognize, due to these studies, that sensitivity to gluten can affect your health even if you're not suffering from celiac disease.

Some of the afflictions that are associated with gluten sensitivity include psoriasis, rheumatoid arthritis, GI upset, fatigue and depression. Scientifically, the links are not fully supported, but physicians who understand the causes for the signs see them all the time. Once patients go gluten-free, even if they did not have diagnosed Celiac disease, their brains begin to function better. They feel fully alive, like someone finally hit the switch on the light and brightened things up.

It was an awakening for many physicians to learn that if people have celiac or simply gluten sensitivity that they are not able to live the same life they could live if they adopted gluten-free diets. It is helpful to choose amaranth, brown rice and quinoa, since they do not have the gluten that may cause you problems.

Using Biomarkers as Signals

There is a discourse among researchers about grains and lectins and their offensive nature. By observing symptoms, physicians can learn how serious the sensitivity to gluten is for their patients. A grain free diet may be required for some patients who have intestinal permeability.

The individuals are studied in stages by their physicians. The diet has to be a manageable one, or the patient will not stay with it. The goal is to get to a point where there is no inflammation in the gut. Gluten sensitivity is still considered dangerous when you don't show celiac in your blood work, but you do have stomach inflammation.

Once the gut is healed, the diet is as manageable as it can be for patients. As long as they do not suffer from Chrohn's disease, colitis or inflammatory bowel disease, they may go back to non-gluten containing grains. If they still develop inflammation, then the physician may pull all the grains from their diet.

Patient Compliance is Vital

If your physician recommends that you go on a gluten-free diet, it is likely that he or she has plenty of information gathered that brings about this decision. Your physician can instruct you to pull all grains from your diet. If you don't adhere to the diet, the symptoms will continue to trouble you.

High performance athletes and others who place their health above all else will usually do what their physicians tell them to do. A gluten-free diet may work well for them. But for everyone with gluten sensitivity to reach their full potential, the masses need to comply.

The gluten-free diet you and your physician choose must be workable. For instance, replacing bread is not something that is easily done. Bakers and brewer's yeast have profound effects on the stomach. This is separate even from the effects of gluten.

It is important for you, as a patient, to understand that you are not giving up gluten just so you won't have stomach problems. You are giving it up so that you will not be more vulnerable to accelerated development of diseases of the immune system.

A recent, published study has shown that if your body is making elevated levels of antibodies to fight the effects of gluten that you will likely develop Chrohn's disease within several years. These are called predictive antibodies. So, if you eat foods with gluten and yeast, your chances of disease are greater.

Beer is also something to be eliminated with a gluten-free diet. It's not enough to cut back on your intake of gluten. You need to cut it out entirely. Otherwise, you may face health issues in the future. This is addressed in "Predictors of Disease" by Abner Notkins at UCLA. It can be found in the March 2006 issue of Scientific American. This can be downloaded at scientificamerican.com.

This article will help you to understand that the mechanisms of disease start much earlier than the symptoms. The mechanisms can be identified and addressed now, in a field known as predictive autoimmunity. This is the issue with sensitivity to gluten.

Other Predictive Health Issue Examples

Women often have thyroid problems even when their thyroid blood tests are normal. This is frustrating, and is similar to the early predictors of celiac disease and gluten sensitivity. Women may have all the signs of thyroid problems without testing positive for thyroid issues:

- Cold extremities
- Low energy levels
- Inability to lose weight even when cutting back on foods

These are all indicators that the thyroid is not functioning properly. Women, especially post partum women, with elevated thyroid antibodies, have over a 90% chance of developing the thyroid disease known as Hashimoto's disease in less than 10 years. This has been proven in published studies. It is recommended that women do not eat gluten before they become pregnant, or during pregnancy.

In Sweden, a report has shown that if a pregnant woman eats gluten, the fetal blood shows autism trends. This was extrapolated in the United States, as well, found at the National Institute of Health. Children who have autism have shown elevated gluten antibodies when they were born.

When the mother has elevated antibodies to gluten in her system, they make it through to her baby, and the baby will be born with an immune response, which is elevated. These children often check positive for autism. This may just be an associated factor. The results were simply observations.

Gluten Effects on the Brain

A recent study that was centered on celiac disease looked into this autoimmune response to gluten. It causes a shortening of the intestinal flora. 73% of people with celiac disease show a lack of proper blood flow to the brain. This is known as hypo perfusion. After a year without gluten in their diet, less than 10% of these people still experienced hypo perfusion.

This problem results when you don't have sufficient blood flowing into your brain. In autistic children, studies show the same behavior patterns, and each is linked to different areas in the brain.

When Are Full Benefits Achieved after Going Gluten-Free?

Once you are not eating any sources of gluten, the time that passes until you become symptom free varies from one individual to the next. It depends on each person, his or her medical history and the amount of damage that had already been done. In many cases, improvement can be seen in as little as three weeks. If you do not feel significantly better in this time, you may want your physician to check for other medical causes for your symptoms.

Many people notice they sleep better after only three or four days of going gluten-free. Their overall outlook is better and their joints don't hurt as they did in the past. Again, it doesn't work if you only reduce your intake. You must cut gluten out of your diet entirely.

You cannot trick your immune system. Your body will always tell you what is going well and what is not. By doing blood work, your physician can tell if you have a problem in your immune system. If your antibodies are elevated, then your immune system is telling you that it has a problem.

Enteric Neural Science Studies

Researchers at Harvard and Stanford have conducted post-doctoral studies regarding enteric neuroscience. This, in short, is the way the stomach affects your brain and your central nervous system. The gut is critical to many of the health concerns you face today. This doesn't mean just stomach pain. It refers to any health concerns that may be related to the stomach.

Colostrum ties into the overall view of health and the stomach. Colostrum has more nutrition within it than any other source. Using that as a basis, you may ask how you can help your gut. If your stomach is inflamed, that must be reduced. This is done by listening to the signals sent by your immune system. If it tells you that there is a problem, then stop eating the foods that cause the problem.

How is the tissue rebuilt after you remove gluten from your diet? In addition, how does your body start production of the proper bacteria that it needs? One ingredient is above all the rest in turning on genes in different ways, and this is colostrum.

Why Is Colostrum so Important?

Colostrum is a mother's first three days of breast milk. When your baby is born and you begin breastfeeding him/her, this is colostrum, not simple breast milk. Colostrum activates the "on" switch in the baby's immune system in the stomach, which starts the production of good bacteria. Enzymes are made that carry messages for more enzymes, to prepare the gut for food. Colostrum is responsible for turning on so many important switches in the gut.

Cow colostrum can be used for children and adults who need those valuable antibodies in their system. Human and cow colostrum show no difference at the molecular level. When you are attempting to heal your stomach, using quality colostrum is a good choice.

The Gluten Free Summit

Researchers who work in the field of celiac disease and gluten sensitivity are eager to share their specific knowledge with others. This will help patients to understand the big picture of gluten sensitivity and how it manifests itself.

Dr. Tom O'Bryan spoke with experts from around the world for the Gluten Summit. The scientists he spoke to are among the leaders in research into celiac disease and gluten sensitivity. He went to Oxford, in England, where he interviewed Michael Marsh, known as "the godfather of celiac diagnosis". Marsh reiterates that any inflammation in the gut is as serious as celiac disease.

Dr. O'Bryan spoke with a number of nutritionists to carry forward the importance of a gluten-free diet for those who have a sensitivity to gluten.

Non-Celiac Gluten Sensitivity

Many people once believed that "using" gluten to explain symptoms was simply reaching for an explanation. However, today's research reveals that this is an actual condition, non-celiac gluten sensitivity (NCGS).

NCGS is not the same as celiac disease; rather, it covers the physical explanations for sensitivities to gluten and the symptoms they create. The people who experience these symptoms may also be sensitive to carbohydrates, which makes treatment more challenging.

Monash University Study, 2011

Dr. Peter Gibson is a gastroenterologist at Monash University in Australia. In 2011, he and several colleagues studied 34 patients who had irritable bowel syndrome (IBS). They did not suffer from celiac disease, but they did have sensitivity to gluten. The study split the group into two, and provided one half with a Gluten-Free diet. After just 3 weeks the Gluten-Free group had seriously reduced symptoms, many showing none at all. The group consuming gluten, as you may expect showed no reduction in symptoms.

Gluten's Effects on the Intestine

Gluten has negative effects on the intestine's barrier function. This allows substances to leak through the intestine into the bloodstream. This was determined in a controlled trial with patients on gluten-free diets, who also have IBS diarrhea effects on intestinal function and bowel frequency. This was published in National Institutes of Health.

IBS involves digestive problems of unknown causes. It affects almost 15% of people in the United States. Some IBS cases may be brought on or exacerbated by gluten. This study was reported in the US National Library of Medicine.

This study makes it clear that even people without gluten sensitivity may react in a negative way to gluten. Other studies, too, show that IBS patients without diagnosed sensitivity to gluten may still have adverse reactions to it.

The Differences between Celiac Disease and NCGS

A Mayo Clinic gastroenterologist, Dr. Joseph A. Murray, is an expert on celiac disease. He states that it is important to be tested for celiac disease before diet changes are made. Celiac disease is much more prevalent in the last 10-20 years than it once was. Gluten sensitivity signs are often similar to those of irritable bowel syndrome and other gastroenterological problems.

Testing first is important, according to Dr. Murray, before the patient goes on a gluten free diet. Once you are on a gluten-free diet, your tests will not allow for an accurate diagnosis.

If you have gluten sensitivity without celiac disease, you will not suffer as much damage to your small intestine. To be sure that you have NCGS, your physician will run tests, to make this determination. The findings may include:

- Improvement in symptoms with removal of gluten from your diet

- Negative tests for celiac disease
- No intestinal damage at biopsy
- Recurrence of the symptoms if gluten is reintroduced
- Symptoms with no other explanation

Once celiac disease is ruled out, your physician can test for non-celiac gluten sensitivity by removing all gluten from your diet for three to four weeks. If your symptoms disappear, begin eating gluten again, to find out whether they will recur. You can also keep a detailed food log for several weeks. This entails recording everything that you eat and drink, along with any symptoms you experience afterwards.

Gluten and Fibromyalgia

Fibromyalgia causes generalized pain, among other symptoms in a broad spectrum. Those who suffer from fibromyalgia may experience cognitive dysfunction, headaches, sleep disturbances and chronic fatigue.

In addition, many fibromyalgia patients have gastrointestinal symptoms that may be overlooked by some studies. A study was conducted in August of 2014 by Mahmoud Slim, Fernando Rico-Villademoros and Elena Pita Calandre from the Instituto de Neurociencias, and was published in Rheumatology

International, regarding the exploration of gastrointestinal aspects of fibromyalgia.

Several studies have discovered that fibromyalgia patients may also experience irritable bowel syndrome (IBS). Other gastrointestinal symptoms included bowel changes, dyspepsia and abdominal pain.

There are several underlying mechanisms that could potentially be at the root of these manifestations. Sensitivity to gluten is one such cause of gastrointestinal symptoms. Study into the links between sensitivity to gluten and the symptoms of fibromyalgia may lead to favorable treatment alternatives.

Why Some Physicians Recommend Going Gluten-Free

Dr. Frank Lipman is the director and founder of 11-11 Wellness Center in New York City. He is a recognized expert in functional and integrative medicine. He often recommends eating plans that have no gluten.

The reason he prescribes this type of eating plan is the presence of specific proteins in gluten that cause the immune system to react as it would to foreign bodies. Gluten, he states, is not well-digested, which is accepted by most physicians and nutritionists.

Most patients who do not have celiac disease have gluten sensitivities. Gluten causes their systems to react in a way that slows them down. This reaction creates inflammation with many effects. They extend to all systems, including the digestive tract, joints, heart and brain.

Physicians are often unable to diagnose gluten sensitivity, since it may present itself as vague unwellness. Gluten can be the cause of many different medical issues, and to treat those, you must treat the sensitivity to gluten.

Many people suffer from gluten intolerance, but are not aware of the fact. Estimates show that about 99% of people who have problems with gluten do not even know that this is what their problem is. Their symptoms often are not specific, and some are not related to their digestive tract.

The serious affects gluten can have on your health are becoming clearer. The more readily it is recognized, the sooner it can be properly treated.

Moving Forward

I hope this chapter has convinced you that gluten is really quite bad for your health. The number of physical and psychological issues that it has been linked to in 1000s of studies is just staggering. These are no small issues either – Autism, depression, crohn's disease, liver cancer, all serious conditions that in some cases are life threatening. The next couple of chapters focus on how to eradicate gluten from your diet so please, please take action here. These studies are all very real.

Chapter Three - How to Make the Transition to Gluten-Free Foods – and Avoid the Common Mistakes!

Gluten-free diets are the main way to treat celiac disease and gluten sensitivity, but this transition can be challenging. You find gluten in so many commercial foods that it can be difficult to eliminate gluten from your diet. In addition, you will want to speak with your physician, and possibly consult a professional dietician, before you make diet changes.

Research the Requirements of Your New Diet

Educate yourself on the foods you will need to leave out of your new diet. Knowing what you can safely eat makes it easier to transition. Concentrate on the foods that you can eat, to begin your healing process.

You can find gluten free foods in your local grocery store, and in specialty stores. They may also be purchased online. Remove the temptation of gluten from your kitchen and replace the foods with healthy, gluten-free alternatives.

Vegetables, greens, eggs, poultry, fish, meat, legumes, seeds, nuts and fruit are naturally free of gluten, as long as they have not been processed, or had something added. Focus on these foods.

Increase your use of these acceptable foods, particularly fruits, greens and veggies, so that you won't suffer from nutrient deprivation. Foods like nuts, seeds, olives, coconut and avocado will keep you from missing your old favorite foods so much. Eating nourishing foods will aid in healing the damage that gluten has caused in your gut.

Major Changes Must Be Made

Whether you have gluten sensitivity or celiac disease, you'll need to make major changes to the way you eat. You may feel at a loss for energy, or experience aches and pains, in addition to stomach issues, so you'll be glad to know that there is a reason for these symptoms. But it can be a bit overwhelming, too.

Your first grocery trip post-diagnosis will probably include hours of wandering aisles and reading labels! Don't worry, you'll get the hang of it. Finding the first few gluten-free versions of foods you love will be exhilarating. After a time, you'll become accustomed to your new diet. If you're still confused, this book will help you to make the transition to healthy, gluten-free foods.

Open Yourself to the New You

Say yes to the new choices in front of you. Sure, it may be difficult to find suitable replacements for the foods you love that are now off-limits. Since your body will not tolerate gluten, eating your old favorites will only make you feel rotten. Store brand hamburger buns or doughnuts are not worth the aftermath.

This is your new life and your new reality. You'll feel so much better without gluten. Accept the new foods you will eat and accept your new life.

Focus on foods that are gluten-free naturally. Sweet potatoes, steaks, salads and raisins are all gluten-free and healthy choices. You will find new foods that you'll love, and you won't go hungry. Don't choose unhealthy gluten foods, or you're missing the point. A calorie laden, gluten-free muffin is still a blueberry muffin. You can find gluten-free junk food, but that's not what you need. Although I will admit these foods did help me make the original transition! Just don't make it a long term habit.

Humans always focus first on things they cannot eat. It's natural. But it's better to think about your health and about the foods you can still eat. You will feel so much better. Some of the foods you love now are gluten-free, so not everything will change. Focus on the positives and eat well.

Cheating Will Make the Transition More Difficult

There will be moments when you're angry and there is no restaurant or store close by that sells the foods you should be eating. When you feel hungry and isolated at the same time, it's quite tempting to eat something that you know is not healthy for you. Don't do it.

It's okay to feel bad once in a while and be angry with your situation. Then you need to move on, with your eyes forward. It won't be perfect, of course. You'll have nights when you have to work late and you come home to nothing healthy in the refrigerator. Go to the pantry, instead. If you've been shopping right, you can still find something for dinner. Going gluten free successfully is about planning ahead.

Inevitably, there will be times when you experience cross-contamination, where gluten comes into contact with the food you eat, usually from equipment used for both types of food. You'll feel it soon after you eat, possibly within minutes. You may start with a headache, but stomach pains won't be far behind. Believe it or not, this is actually how you felt constantly whilst consuming gluten regularly. The way you feel after that is over will be more than adequate to remind you why you cannot eat gluten any longer.

Are You a Cook? You Will Be

If you already cook, you may enjoy the challenge of creating new dishes. Listening to the sounds of cooking and smelling the aromas is enjoyable. If you didn't cook before you were diagnosed with gluten sensitivity or celiac disease, you probably will afterward.

Cooking will be a path to healing. You may be hesitant to allow others to cook for you, after experiences of cross-contamination. You may learn to cook and you will probably become quite adept at creating meals that your whole family will enjoy.

Even if you're not competent cooking before now, you will become accustomed to chopping and cleaning vegetables and taking the time to use new recipes. Cooking can become a means of concentration and you will focus on the foods before you. You can use cooking to ease the stress of the day away.

Perhaps you're thinking that you don't have time to take up cooking, since your life is busy. Take another look at the idea.

Eating foods that you know are gluten-free is your singular path to healing. Your entire life will change, and it will be a positive change. Simply arrange your life a bit differently so that you'll have time to cook.

People on Your Side

It's always good to have people on your side, and this will be particularly true now. Your significant other or a close friend can help you with the cooking aspects of a non-gluten lifestyle. Together, you can find recipes on which to work, and your friends can cheer you up through the process.

If your kitchen still has gluten breads, pastas and cereals, it may be more difficult for you to make the new diet work. If your husband or wife and children don't want to share your road to gluten-free eating, have them try it just for a week. Cook your best non-gluten dishes and see if you can win them over. Then you won't have to worry about cross-contamination.

If you choose to eat gluten-free food in cafes or restaurants, be sure to patronize those that will not cross-contaminate your food. You may lose weight if you eat at places with cross-contamination, but your gut will certainly not thank you.

You need a solid community with you, including friends who will understand the changes you will be making, and a family who will support you. There will even be those who are there for you when you need to cry a little because someone wonders insensitively how a little flour could hurt you.

There are many support rooms where you can find people in similar situations, including forums, chat rooms and local groups. Seek out people who will let you know that you are not alone in this journey. Soon your body will thank you for the change, and you will feel so much better.

Be Patient with Yourself during the Transition

Show yourself compassion and love as you adjust to your new lifestyle. Food is an integral part of culture. When your food choices change, especially due to your health, you can feel out of sorts for a time, as your body adjusts. Give yourself extra care by going for walks, talking to old friends, getting a massage or going out dancing. Keeping a journal is helpful, so that you can note how you feel and what your energy level is like after you eat certain foods. This journal tracks what foods help you and what foods do not.

Plan Ahead for Your Meals

Prepare a list of foods you will use for meals and take it with you to the grocery store. When you arrive home, wash, cut up and prepare your foods so they will be ready to eat when you need them. This will make your new food routine easier.

Whenever you cook, make enough for leftovers and then stock your freezer with ready-to-heat meals. This will make it easier to prepare meals after a long day at work. Stock your house with tasty new foods and get rid of old foods that might otherwise tempt you. Keep the fixings for meals and healthy snacks available at home, so you won't go out or call out for meals.

Eat Fewer Meals Out and More at Home

When you eat out, there is no easy way to see the ingredients used in preparing your meals. If you just have to have a meal out, call ahead of time and find restaurants that have choices including gluten free meals. When you are eating out, ask your server before you order a dish.

If your server is new or not knowledgeable about the foods used, you can speak to a manager. Always be polite to food service employees, while still being assertive about the types of foods you need. Thank them and let them know that you appreciate their help. This will make them more willing to help others who are also making the transition to gluten-free foods.

If you didn't know how to cook before, you will need to, now. This doesn't mean you have to cook well enough to win a TV show. You just need to be able to fix yourself meals that are nourishing. As you discover new cuisines and recipes, you may find that you enjoy cooking.

Keep Healthy Snacks Available

Take snacks to work with you and eat a healthy meal before you head out anywhere. Keeping foods you can snack on will stop you from eating foods that contain gluten. Substitutions make it much easier to transition to new foods, especially at the beginning.

Gluten-free bread and other foods will make it simpler to ease into your new menu. Select substitutions that are minimally processed and high in nutritive value. Read the labels on every type of food, before you make your purchases.

Gluten may be hidden in many products that you would not suspect. Gluten is even found in some body products like toothpaste!

Once you get used to reading labels, it will be easier for you, since you'll know what you're looking to find. Experiment with new foods, and consult your nutritionist to determine the best food choices for you.

Celebrate with the foods you can still eat. Gluten-free diets may seem restrictive when you first take them on, but there are many things you will still be able to enjoy. Unprocessed foods are the best, so avoid seasoned, breaded and marinated items, since they may contain gluten.

Learning the Safe Grains

There are grains you can still eat on a gluten-free diet. You can eat some carbohydrates. Tapioca, soy, sorghum, rice, quinoa, millet, flax, corn, buckwheat, arrowroot and amaranth are all among the grains you can still enjoy.

Use gluten-free flours, too. You may decide that you enjoy muffins, cookies and bread made with nut, potato or bean flour. You can adapt your own flour-centered recipes with gluten-free alternatives.

Remember the Foods to Avoid

Stay clear of foods that might give you problems, unless you see on their labels that they are gluten-free. Products that often contain gluten may include a wide variety of foods like seasoned vegetables, soup, snacks, seasoned rice mix, condiments, imitation seafood, lunch meats, gravy, French fries, bread, candy, baked goods and crackers.

Remember the grains you need to avoid, as well. Reading the labels is quite important. The grains you should not eat anymore include spelt, semolina, kamut, graham, durum, bulgur, farina, triticale, rye, wheat and barley.

Diversification of tastes will necessitate that you lose the local listings of Italian restaurants, since their pizzas and rich pastas will cause your stomach to react. Indian cooking is often better, and so are yogurt, legumes, rice and chickpeas.

A Stroll through the Grocery Store

After you take in everything in your local store that is gluten-free, you might be thinking that it would be better for everyone to be on a gluten-free diet. Staying away from gluten-free cakes, cookies and other types of junk foods is a healthy way to eat, even if someone doesn't have gluten insensitivity or celiac disease.

Millions of people avoid the gluten found in wheat, rye and barley, to help them in losing weight or to create less stomach distress.

Gluten-Free Food Distributors

Whole Foods Markets have an entire line of sweets that are gluten-free. That doesn't mean that gluten-free sweets are any better for you than conventional kinds in conventional healthy measures. They can be used as a reward for having a successful week free of gluten though!

Glutino offers gluten-free cookies, pretzels, toaster pastries and baked potato crisps. You won't lose weight with gluten-free sweets, but once in awhile you need to think of your sweet tooth.

Chapter Four – Great, Healthy Gluten-Free Diet Planning

Eating a diet that is free of gluten will help you to control your symptoms and signs of celiac disease or gluten sensitivity, and prevent any complications. You may be initially frustrated at the prospect of a gluten-free diet, but with time and creativity, you'll discover many foods that are gluten-free and still quite tasty.

Switching is a Big Change

Switching to a healthy, gluten-free diet isn't a small change. As with anything new, you will need to become accustomed to your diet options. There are more gluten-free food choices than ever available at groceries and health food stores. Be sure to speak with a registered dietician, so that you know what type of diet plan will suit you.

What Can You Eat?

Your dining plan includes many delicious and healthy foods that are still allowed. Some are naturally gluten-free, like:
- Fresh eggs
- Unprocessed nuts, seeds and beans

- Fresh poultry, meat and fish (not marinated, breaded or batter-coated)
- Most types of dairy products
- Vegetables and fruits

Be sure to choose foods that are not mixed or processed with preservatives, grains or additives that contain gluten. Many starches and grains have a place in a gluten-free diet.

Baking without Gluten

If baking is a type of chemistry, then baking without gluten is a science. Your first few times baking without using gluten may be somewhat disheartening. Muffins can be hard, and cakes may be listless. Don't give up hope though, I honestly think a good gluten free cake is stunningly tasty. It's a really impressive skill to work on and master.

The Power of Flour

You will learn to create your own baking mixes with gluten-free flour. If you are hungry for muffins, consider using whole-grain sorghum, millet and brown rice. If you're making cookies, you may want them to be crunchy and crisp. Potato starch and tapioca work well here. There is plenty of information about gluten free flours on the internet, honestly I could write an entire book about them. A quick search on google will provide you with all the answers you need, regarding baking and flour.

Texture is Important

All-purpose flour has different textures of flours within it. You will want to replicate that idea without using wheat, barley or rye. Blend in other, gluten-free flours, to get the taste and texture you prefer. Rice flour, for example, gives your baked goods a powdery quality.

Serious bakers will weigh the ingredients, including flour, to get the proportions right. If you don't have time for that, you can use all-purpose flour mixes that are gluten-free.

Working on Elasticity

Gluten gives baked goods their stickiness. You'll need to replicate this without gluten. To do this, you may use guar gum and xanthan gum to give your batter and dough the stretchy, pliable quality they need to bake into tender or crispy morsels. These gums are available in powder versions, and they stabilize, thicken and emulsify recipes. Some gluten-free all-purpose flours already include guar gum or xanthan gum. It's good to remember that many foods that are gluten-free have a shorter shelf life, so don't stock up on a lot more than you will be needing in the near future. In addition, homemade foods should be consumed sooner than usual, because they are missing some stabilizers and preservatives.

The Cost of Going Gluten-Free

Gluten-free baking has an upfront investment involved. You may want up to four or five different flours in your pantry. Otherwise, the things you bake will feel and taste the same. Use airtight containers in which to store your gluten-free ingredients. If you don't bake often, freeze or refrigerate the flour, so that it won't spoil. You can often get the best prices on gluten free foods if you buy online. However, you may find that cooking and baking from scratch is even more affordable than buying gluten-free foods ready-made.

Read those Labels

With the recently increasing interest in a gluten-free diets, many new products are on the grocery shelves. Do pay attention to labels. Some foods are emblazoned with "no gluten ingredients". This isn't the same as "gluten-free" foods. Read labels very carefully, and find brands that you trust to be gluten-free. Pay attention to the products you buy on a regular basis. If you develop symptoms from something, toss it, and don't buy any more.

Gluten-Free Baking Tips

Store gluten-free, moist baked goods in containers that are airtight. Otherwise they may dry out more quickly. If you read "modified food starch" on a label, contact the product manufacturer to find out whether the starch is from corn, or other gluten-free products. Not every food you want has a gluten-free option. You can usually find gluten-free alternatives online, if you don't have them available locally.

Cross-Contamination Concerns

You may consume gluten at some time without knowing it. Gluten is found in sources where you wouldn't expect it, like in meat products, pharmaceuticals or confectionary desserts. If you don't prepare your own foods, you will run into cross-contamination, eventually. Cross-contamination occurs more often at parties or social events, when eating out and when you travel. You will need to make sure you let your host know about your new diet. If you are not confident that they will be able to adhere to your restrictions then politely request that you bring some of your own food. Explain it is for medicinal purposes and is definitely not an insult to them! Most people will fully understand.

Take Your Vitamins

If you eat a gluten free diet, you may not get enough vitamins in the foods you eat. Grains that you no longer eat are vitamin-enriched, so avoiding those may mean that you don't get as many enriched foods. If you are eating a diet rich in fruits and vegetables this probably won't be a concern. Speak with your

dietician about supplementing, if you need to, so that you get enough:
- Calcium
- Iron
- Fiber
- Riboflavin
- Thiamin
- Folate
- Niacin

Even if you don't experience abdominal issues when you accidentally eat a product with gluten in it, it is still damaging your intestines. Trace gluten amounts can cause damage, without symptoms. Other common deficiencies in gluten-free diets are Vitamins A, K, D and E, phosphorous and B12. Eating high protein foods is helpful, to avoid malnutrition.

What to Look for on Food Packaging
Wheat-free does not mean gluten-free. Read your ingredients lists.

Fillers with gluten are sometimes used in medications. Ask your pharmacist and check the labels to be sure that they do not contain gluten. Contacting the company that manufactures the medication will also yield the answer.

When you are using foods with gluten for your family, be careful to avoid cross-contamination. Just putting a non-gluten ingredient into a bowl that contained gluten risks cross-contamination. There are other ways cross-contamination may occur, as well. They include:

Toasters or toaster ovens – use separate units for gluten-free foods

Crumbs left in butter, jelly or condiments – use squeezable containers

Double Dipping – be sure that people don't stick utensils or foods in any of your gluten-free foods, like hummus or butter

Storage – make separate spaces in the refrigerator and cabinets

Foods You Can Consume on a Gluten-Free Diet

There used to be a very limited number of gluten-free foods available. Today, you have more choices than ever before, and the list of foods is growing.

Safe foods include:

- Arrowroot
- Amaranth
- Buckwheat
- Bread made with potato flour or rice flour
- Corn
- Chestnuts
- Flax
- Distilled vinegar
- Grits (soy or corn)
- Garbanzo beans (also known as chickpeas)

- Hominy
- Herbs
- Lentils
- Nut flours
- Millet
- Pumpkin
- Potatoes
- Rice
- Quinoa
- Seeds
- Sago
- Sorghum
- Soy
- Teff
- Tapioca

Other foods you can eat on your gluten-free diet include:
- Meats for protein
- Dry beans and peas, soybeans, peanut butter and nuts
- Plain eggs, shellfish, fish and poultry
- Fruit
- Tofu
- Fruit juice
- Fruits

- Canned, fresh and frozen vegetables
- Dairy foods
- Cottage cheese
- Plain yogurt
- Cheese

Beverages

- Ground or pure instant coffee
- Carbonated beverages
- Tea
- Beer made from corn, rice, sorghum or buckwheat- Be careful here and read the label.
- Alcohol including wine, vodka, tequila, rum, gin, champagne, brandy – Be careful here as well, plenty of brands do now include gluten in their alcohol.

Fats

- Margarine
- Butter
- Lard
- Vegetable oils

Gluten Is Sneaky

You can find hidden gluten in many sources you might not expect, including:

- Tamari-style stir fry sauce
- Soy sauce
- Gravy
- Marinades
- Bouillon
- Broth
- Instant soups
- Cooking sauces
- Cured meat
- Salad dressing
- Hot dogs
- Sausage
- Vegan hot dogs
- Burgers
- Herb and flavored cheese
- Dry mustard
- Curry powder and other spice blends

Be sure that you always read labels on products, to make sure that gluten was not used in their production. This includes:

- Tomato paste
- Prepared and canned soups
- Confectioner's sugars

- Sweeteners
- Instant and flavored coffees
- Prepared beverages
- Herbal teas (look for barley in the ingredients)
- Jerky
- Spiced, roasted or flavored nuts
- Flavored yogurts
- Ice cream
- Pudding
- Chocolate
- Instant cocoa mix
- Cocoa powder
- Flavored vinegars
- Malt wine coolers
- Flavored liquers
- Cooking wines

Eating Out is Tricky

Eating out can be quite tricky if you're trying to eat gluten-free. Restaurants and delis may add pancake mix or flour to omelets, and they may use breadcrumbs to give extra body to things like tuna salad.

Gluten-free pasta sounds safe, doesn't it? What if it's boiled in the water that was previously used for standard types of pasta? That causes cross-contamination. Avoid fried foods and French fries made in the same oil as breaded, gluten-filled foods like batter coated fish, chicken and meat or fried onion rings.

Be sure to check reviews for restaurants online or engage in gluten free groups to find out which restaurants are the best suited for you. There are now entire restaurants that are strictly free, if you are nearby one of these then you have hit the gold mine!

Baking and Cooking Gluten-Free

After a time, cooking safely will become second nature to you. Safe flours for gluten-free baking include

- Teff flour
- Quinoa flour
- Buckwheat flour
- Millet flour
- Sweet rice flour
- White rice flour
- Brown rice flour
- Sorghum flour
- Oat flour that is certified to be gluten-free.

Some starches you can use for baking gluten-free include tapioca flour or starch, arrowroot starch, cornstarch and potato starch. You can use coconut flour to add texture, flavor and moisture to gluten-free foods.

If you're new to gluten-free baking, try Pamela's Ultimate Pancake and Baking Mix for your recipes. This is pre-mixed and ready to use for simple cakes, muffins and tea breads. It also works quite well for pancakes, flour-less quiches and omelets. It does have buttermilk in its recipe, so it's not for those on dairy-free diets.

Gluten-Free Baking Tips

Number One: Keep a healthy sense of humor. It will help in baking with gluten-free ingredients. Doorstops and hockey pucks are to be expected. Toss them and try again.

Gluten-free, all-purpose flour is not always the best choice for baking gluten free treats. Many of these have rice flour as a base, since it is inexpensive to make. The result is a bland baked item, and the flavor and texture leave something to be desired.

If you can tell that your baking goods are gluten-free, try not using precise "cup for a cup" measurements of all-purpose flours. It can make them gritty or gummy. Bean flours don't work exceptionally well for sweets, either.

Some new all-purpose, gluten-free flour blends have better results, but this is usually due to their inclusion of buttermilk or milk powder in the blend. If you're reactive to dairy, that won't work for you.

Diet Plans

Once you have in mind your favorite gluten-free foods, plan your meals at least a week out. Divide your days into three main meals with healthy snacks or five to six smaller meals. I won't post a specific diet plan here, since it would not include the foods you like and will personally want to include.

Post your plan on your refrigerator so it's easy to use. You'll find that gluten free eating doesn't have to be a hassle.

10 Delicious Gluten Free Breakfast Recipes

GLUTEN FREE PANCAKES

YIELD: 4 SERVINGS

INGREDIENTS:
- 1/2 a cup of almond flour
- 1/4 cup of buckwheat flour
- 1 1/4 cup of sorghum flour
- 1/4 cup of potato starch
- 1 teaspoon of salt
- 1 teaspoon of xanthan gum
- 2 teaspoons of baking powder
- 1 cup of water
- 1 cup of soy milk
- 2 eggs, beaten
- 3 tablespoons of coconut oil
- 1 tablespoon of honey
- 1 teaspoon of pure vanilla extract
- 1 teaspoon of almond extract

DIRECTIONS:
- Heat a large pan on medium heat and grease if required.
- Whisk together in a large mixing bowl all the dry ingredients.
- Make a well in the center.
- Mix together in a separate large bowl all the wet ingredients.

- Slowly add the wet ingredients to the dry ingredients and beat well to combine.
- Your batter should not be too thick but silky and smooth.
- Use a ladle and pour a scoop of the pancake batter onto the heated pan, repeat this for as many pancakes as you can fit into your pan.
- Wait for tiny bubbles to appear on your pancakes and then flip them over with a spatula.
- Only cook them for a minute or two as you do not want to overcook the pancakes as they will become tough.
- Eat them straight away with maple syrup.
- Alternatively you can add some fresh fruit to your batter before cooking them, such as some fresh blueberries, bananas etc.

SCRAMBLED TOFU

This recipe can be served with your choice of fresh vegetables to add to it, such as mushrooms, green peppers, onions etc.

YIELD: 2 SERVINGS

INGREDIENTS:
- 1 box of silken tofu
- 2 tablespoons of olive oil for the pan
- Salt and pepper to taste

DIRECTIONS:
- Add the tofu into a medium sized saucepan and add water to just cover the tofu.
- Bring it to a boil and let it simmer for around 10 minutes.
- Drain the water from the tofu.
- Transfer to a place and cut the tofu into bite size pieces.
- Place a pan on a medium heat and add in the olive oil and heat up.
- Add pieces of the tofu to the frying pan and season well.
- Cook until the tofu is a lovely golden brown.
- Add in any vegetables of your choice.
- Serve warm.

CINNAMON QUINOA PORRIDGE

YIELD: 1 SERVING

INGREDIENTS:
- 1/4 of a cup of quinoa flakes
- 1 teaspoon of cinnamon
- 1/2 a teaspoon of ginger
- 1/2 a teaspoon of nutmeg
- 1 tablespoon of vanilla extract
- 1 cup of almond milk
- 4 dried pruned, chopped
- 1 tablespoon of maple syrup
- 1/2 a tablespoon of raw sliced almonds

DIRECTIONS:
- In a pot on a medium heat, bring the almond milk to a boil.
- Add in the quinoa flakes and cook for 30 seconds, stirring frequently.
- Add in the ginger, vanilla, cinnamon, prunes and nutmeg and combine well.
- Cook for another 30 seconds while continuing to stir.
- Remove from the heat and allow to cool.
- Add in the maple syrup and sprinkle with the almonds.

BAKED EGGS IN A PORTOBELLO MUSHROOM

YIELD: 4 SERVINGS

INGREDIENTS:
- 4 eggs
- 4 large Portobello mushroom caps
- 4 slices of prosciutto
- Salt and pepper to taste
- Fresh parsley
- A little olive oil

DIRECTIONS:
- Preheat the oven to 180C degrees.
- Clean the Portobello mushroom caps with a clean damp cloth and remove the stem.
- Scrape out the gills so that you have a nice well that is deep enough for the egg.
- Rub a little olive oil onto the outside of the mushrooms to help it to cook and to keep it from sticking to the pan.
- Arrange the mushrooms onto a baking sheet.
- Place a slice of prosciutto inside of the mushroom cap and then carefully crack an egg onto each slice of prosciutto.
- Sprinkle each one with salt and pepper and the chopped parsley. Do not add too much salt as the prosciutto is already salty.
- Carefully place the baking tray in the pre-heated oven.
- Bake for 25 - 30 minutes.

VERY BERRY OMLETTE

YIELD: 1 SERVING

INGREDIENTS:
- 1 large egg
- 100g of cottage cheese
- 180g of chopped blueberries, raspberries and strawberries
- 2 tablespoon of skimmed milk
- 1 teaspoon of cinnamon
- 1 tablespoon of olive oil

DIRECTIONS:
- In a mixing bowl, beat the milk, eggs and cinnamon together.
- Heat a large non-stick frying pan with olive oil.
- Pour in the egg mixture and make sure that it covers the base of the pan.
- Cook for a couple of minutes until it has set and is golden underneath.
- You do not need to flip it over.
- Place on a serving plate and spread the cottage cheese over the omelet.
- Scatter with berries.
- Roll it up and serve.

BAKED FRUITS WITH VANILLA

YIELD: 4 SERVINGS

INGREDIENTS:
- 1 vanilla pod, split in two
- 165g golden caster sugar
- 4 cardamom pods
- 6 apricots, halved and stoned
- 3 peaches, quartered and stoned
- 3 nectarines, quartered and stoned
- Zest and juice of 1 lime

DIRECTIONS:
- Heat the oven to 220C degrees.
- In a food processor, add the vanilla pod, cardamom, sugar and lemon juice and blitz until well blended.
- Add the fruit into a shallow baking dish.
- Toss in the sugar mixture and coat the fruit evenly.
- Place in the pre-heated oven for 25 minutes, the fruits should all be soft.
- The juice will be nice and sticky.
- Serve with some Greek Yoghurt.

SPICY TOMATO BAKED EGGS

YIELD: 2 SERVINGS

INGREDIENTS:
- 2 red onions, chopped
- 1 garlic clove, crushed
- 1 chili, deseeded and chopped
- 1 can of cherry tomatoes
- 1 tablespoon of caster sugar
- 1 tablespoon of olive oil
- 4 eggs

DIRECTIONS:
- In a large frying pan that has a lid, heat the olive oil on a medium heat.
- Add in the onions, chili and garlic and gently cook until soft.
- Stir in the tomatoes and the sugar and let it simmer for 10 minutes.
- Make 4 dips in the sauce by using the back of a spoon.
- Gently crack an egg into each dip.
- Place a lid on the pan and cook on a low heat until the eggs are done to your liking.

ORANGE POLENTA

YIELD: 4 SERVINGS

INGREDIENTS:
- 3/4 of a cup of instant polenta
- 1 orange
- 2 cups of water
- 1 cup of skimmed milk
- 1/4 cup of mascarpone cheese
- 1/4 cup of Greek Yoghurt
- 4 tablespoons of honey
- A pinch of salt

DIRECTIONS:
- Grate the orange peel and set the zest aside.
- Cut the segments from the remaining orange and set aside.
- In a saucepan over a medium heat, combine the water, milk and salt and bring to a boil.
- Whisk in the polenta gradually and bring it to the boil.
- Reduce the heat to low and cook for around 5 minutes.
- Remove from the heat and let it rest for 5 minutes.
- In a separate mixing bowl, combine the mascarpone, 1 tablespoon of honey, orange zest and yoghurt.
- Whisk the remaining 3 tablespoons of honey into the polenta.
- Divide among 4 bowl and then top with the mascarpone topping.
- Garnish with the remaining orange segments.

CRISPY POTATOES WITH GREEN BEANS AND EGGS

YIELD: 4 SERVINGS

INGREDIENTS:
- 1/2 a cup of cooked green beans, cut into pieces
- 2 pounds of boiled potatoes, cut into pieces
- 1 garlic clove, crushed
- 1/2 a teaspoon of salt
- Freshly ground pepper to taste
- 4 large eggs
- 2 tablespoons of olive oil

DIRECTIONS:
- In a large frying pan, heat the oil on a medium heat.
- Spread the potatoes in an even layer and cook them turning every few minutes until nicely browned.
- Stir in the green beans, garlic and salt and pepper.
- Gently crack the eggs one at a time over the vegetables.
- Cover with a lid and let the eggs cook.
- Sprinkle the eggs with salt and pepper if desired and serve immediately.

CREAMY BANANA BUCKWHEAT PORRIDGE

YIELD: 2 SERVINGS

INGREDIENTS:
- 1 cup of buckwheat
- 2 cups of almond milk
- 1 cup of water
- 2 bananas
- 1 tablespoon of pure honey
- 1 teaspoon of cinnamon
- 1 tablespoon of almond butter
- 1 tablespoon of baobab powder

DIRECTIONS:
- Place the buckwheat into a pan with boiling water and allow to heat for a couple of minutes.
- Stir in the sliced bananas, honey and cinnamon.
- When the water has been absorbed add in a cup of the almond milk.
- Allow this to keep cooking and then gradually add in the second cup of almond milk.
- The whole meal should take around 20 minutes to cook.
- Stir in the almond butter and the baobab.
- Serve warm.

10 Delicious Gluten Free Lunch Recipes

SPICY TUNA POTATO

YIELD: 1 SERVING

INGREDIENTS:
- 1 can of tuna, drained
- 1 chili, chopped
- 1 spring onion, sliced
- 8 cherry tomatoes, halved
- 1 jacket potato
- 150g cottage cheese
- A handful of fresh coriander, chopped

DIRECTIONS:
- Preheat the oven to 190C degrees.
- Prick the potato with a fork several times.
- Place the potato in the oven and bake for 1 hour or until soft inside.
- In a mixing bowl, combine the tuna, cherry tomatoes, spring onion and coriander together.
- Split the cooked potato open and spoon in the tuna mix.
- Add cottage cheese on top of the tuna mix.
- Serve warm.

CHICKEN CAESAR SALAD

YIELD: 4 SERVINGS

INGREDIENTS:
- 4 skinless chicken breasts
- 1 Cos Lettuce, chopped
- 1 punnet of salad cress
- 3 hardboiled eggs, peeled and halved
- 30g of Parmesan cheese, finely grated
- 50g of anchovies fillets, chopped
- 170g Greek yoghurt
- 2 tablespoons of olive oil
- Juice of 1 lemon

DIRECTIONS:
- Place the chicken breasts in a bowl and add the olive oil and 1 tablespoon of the lemon juice, season with salt and pepper.
- Cook the chicken breasts under the grill for 10 - 15 minutes until cooked through.
- Transfer the chicken to a board and slice when cooked.
- Arrange the lettuce, salad cress and the eggs on a serving platter and then top with the cooked chicken.
- Mix together the Parmesan, anchovies, remaining lemon juice and the yoghurt and season to taste.
- Pour this mixture over the chicken and lettuce.
- Serve

POTATO, LEEK AND PARMESAN FRITATTA

YIELD: 8 SERVINGS

INGREDIENTS:
- 5 leeks, rinsed and sliced into 1/4 inch thick rounds
- 1 pound of potatoes, peeled and cut into cubes
- 8 eggs plus 2 egg whites
- 1 cup of water
- 1 teaspoon of cayenne pepper
- 3/4 cup of ricotta cheese
- 3/4 cup of Parmesan cheese
- 2 cloves of garlic, thinly sliced
- Salt and pepper to taste
- 1 teaspoon of olive oil

DIRECTIONS:
- Preheat the oven to 180C degrees.
- Grease a square baking dish with the olive oil.
- In a medium sized saucepan over a medium heat, bring the water to the boil.
- Add the potatoes, leeks and garlic and season with salt, reduce the heat to low and cook with a lid on until the potatoes are tender.
- Remove from the heat and let them cool down.
- In a mixing bowl whisk together the eggs and the egg whites, season with salt and add in the cayenne pepper.
- Fold the eggs into the potato mixture and add in the ricotta and Parmesan cheese.
- Pour the mixture into the prepared dish and place in the oven and cook for 25 minutes.

- Let the dish cool for 10 minutes before cutting into squares and serving.

BUCKWHEAT NOODLE SALAD WITH CHICKEN AND SCALLIONS

YIELD: 4 SERVINGS

INGREDIENTS:
- 3/4 pounds of buckwheat noodles
- 1/3 cup of gluten free soy sauce
- 3 tablespoons of rice vinegar
- 1 teaspoon of sugar
- 1 tablespoon of olive oil
- 1 garlic clove, crushed
- 1 teaspoon of freshly grated ginger
- 3/4 pounds of cooked chicken, shredded
- 6 scallions, slice thin
- 2 1/2 cups of red cabbage, thinly sliced

DIRECTIONS:
- Cook the buckwheat noodles according to the package instructions and set aside.
- In a large mixing bowl, combine the soy sauce, rice vinegar, sugar, oil, ginger and the garlic together.
- Toss the buckwheat noodles with the soy mixture until evenly coated.
- Add in the shredded chicken, cabbage and scallions, mix well.
- Serve.

SPICY BUTTERNUT AND APPLE SOUP

YIELD: 6 SERVINGS

INGREDIENTS:
- 4 cups of butternut, peeled and chopped
- 1 large apple, peeled and quartered
- 2 carrots, peeled and chopped
- 1 onion, peeled and chopped
- 2 tablespoons of olive oil
- A dash of ground cloves
- 2 garlic cloves, chopped
- 1/2 a teaspoon of turmeric
- 1/2 a teaspoon of cinnamon
- 1/2 a teaspoon of cardamom
- Salt and pepper to taste
- 3 cups of water

DIRECTIONS:
- In a large saucepan on a medium heat, heat the olive oil.
- Add in the garlic and onions and cook until tender.
- Add in the turmeric, cinnamon, cardamom, cloves and ginger and cook until fragrant.
- Add in the carrots, apples and butternut and 3 cups of water and bring to the boil.
- Reduce the heat and let it simmer for 20 minutes, until all the vegetables are tender.
- Season with salt and pepper.
- Blitz the soup in a blender.

MINTY CARROT AND FETA SALAD

YIELD: 6 SERVINGS

INGREDIENTS:
- 500g of carrots, halved and cut into chunks
- 1 can of chickpeas, drained and rinsed
- 2 handfuls of fresh spinach
- 200g of feta cheese, crumbled
- 1 tablespoon of honey
- 2 tablespoons of olive oil
- Juice of 1 lemon
- 1 small handful of fresh mint, chopped
- 1 teaspoon of ground cumin
- 100g of pistachios, roughly chopped

DIRECTIONS:
- Preheat the oven to 180C degrees.
- In a large baking tray, add the carrots, chickpeas and the cumin and season with the olive oil and salt and pepper.
- Place the tray in the oven and cook for 30 minutes, until the carrots are tender.
- Mix together the lemon juice, honey and olive oil and then pour over the cooked carrots. Set aside and leave to cool
- Once the carrot mixture has cooled you can mix in the mint and spinach leaves. Add in the pistachios and scatter the feta.
- Season with salt and pepper if needed and you can drizzle a little extra olive oil on the top.

SPICED QUINOA WITH ALMONDS AND FETA

YIELD: 4 SERVINGS

INGREDIENTS:
- 300g of quinoa, rinsed
- 100g of feta cheese, crumbled
- 60g of toasted flaked almonds
- 1 teaspoon of ground coriander
- 1 teaspoon of turmeric
- Juice of 1 lemon
- 600ml of boiling water
- 1 tablespoon of olive oil
- Salt and pepper to taste

DIRECTIONS:
- In a large pan on a medium heat, heat the olive oil.
- Add all the spices and fry until they are fragrant.
- Add in the rinsed quinoa and fry until you can hear popping sounds.
- Stir in the boiling water and gently simmer for 15 minutes, the water must evaporated.
- Allow to cool slightly, add in all the remaining ingredients and gently mix until all combined.
- Can be served warm or cold.

SWEET POTATO WITH RICOTTA AND KALE

YIELD: 4 SERVINGS

INGREDIENTS:
- 4 sweet potatoes
- 2 garlic cloves, peeled and sliced
- 1 bunch of kale, remove the stems and break the leaves into pieces
- 1 cup of ricotta cheese
- 2 tablespoons of balsamic vinegar
- 3 tablespoons of olive oil
- Seasoning to taste

DIRECTIONS:
- Preheat the oven to 180C degrees.
- Place the sweet potatoes on a baking tray.
- Rub olive oil all over the sweet potatoes to help them cook and not stick to the baking tray.
- Bake the sweet potatoes for 45 minutes to 1 hour, until they are soft inside.
- In a large frying pan, on a medium to high heat, add in a tablespoon of olive oil and fry the garlic until golden, transfer to a paper towel and let it drain.
- Add the kale to the frying pan and season with salt and pepper, cook tossing them frequently until they are tender, around 5 minutes.
- Stir in the vinegar and season with salt and pepper.
- Open each of the sweet potatoes, season with salt and pepper.
- Top the sweet potatoes with the kale and then top with the ricotta cheese.

AVOCADO WITH A BLACK BEAN SALSA

YIELD: 2 SERVINGS

INGREDIENTS:
- 1 large avocado, pitted
- 3 lime wedges
- 2 tomatoes, chopped into cubes
- 1 red onion, peeled and diced
- 4 tablespoons of black beans, drained
- Salt and Pepper to taste
- 1 tablespoon of olive oil

DIRECTIONS:
- Season the avocado halves with salt and squeeze with the limes.
- In a separate bowl, combine the tomatoes, onions, black beans and olive oil and season with salt and pepper.
- Top this mixture onto the halved avocados.
- Serve.

RICE NOODLES WITH A BROCCOLI AND ALMOND PESTO

YIELD: 4 SERVINGS

INGREDIENTS:
- 1 head of broccoli, broken up
- 8 tablespoons of toasted almonds, sliced
- 1/2 a cup of fresh basil leaves
- 2 garlic cloves, crushed
- 2 tablespoons of lemon juice
- 1 packet of rice noodles
- 4 tablespoons of olive oil
- Salt and pepper to taste

DIRECTIONS:
- Cook the rice noodles according to the packet instructions, drain and set aside.
- Steam the broccoli florets until they are just tender and let them cool down slightly.
- Roughly chop up about 1 cup of the broccoli and set aside.
- In a blender, blend the remaining broccoli, almonds, basil, garlic and the lemon juice.
- Add in the olive oil to the pesto mix and season with salt and pepper.
- Toss the broccoli pieces together with the rice noodles.
- Gently stir through your pesto mix and season with salt and pepper.
- Serve.

10 Delicious Gluten Free Dinner Recipes

ORANGE AND HONEY SEA BASS WITH LENTILS

YIELD: 2 SERVINGS

INGREDIENTS:
- 2 large sea bass fillets
- 250g or lentils, cooked
- 100g of watercress
- Juice and Zest of 1 orange
- 2 tablespoons of honey
- 2 tablespoons of olive oil
- 2 tablespoons of wholegrain mustard
- A bunch of fresh parsley, chopped
- A bunch of fresh dill, chopped

DIRECTIONS:
- Preheat the oven to 180C degrees.
- Line a baking tray with foil and place the sea bass, skin side down, on the foil.
- In a separate bowl, combine the orange zest, mustard, honey and olive oil. Season well with salt and pepper.
- Drizzle this mixture over the sea bass and pull the sides of the foil up to make a parcel.
- Place in the preheated oven and bake for 15 minutes.
- Warm the lentils and mix with the orange juice and a tablespoon of olive oil, add in the watercress, fresh herbs and season.

- Divide the lentils between two plates and top each plate with the cooked sea bass, drizzle over the juices that are left from roasting the sea bass.
- Serve immediately.

SHERRY CHICKEN WITH ALMONDS AND DATES

YIELD: 4 SERVINGS

INGREDIENTS:
- 8 chicken legs
- 2 onions, roughly chopped
- 12 garlic cloves, left whole in the skin
- 250ml of sherry
- Juice and Zest of 1 lemon
- 60g of whole blanched almonds, roughly chopped
- 10 soft dates, chopped
- 1 teaspoon of ground cumin
- 3 tablespoons of olive oil

DIRECTIONS:
- Preheat the oven to 200C degrees.
- In a large frying pan, over a medium to high heat, heat the olive oil.
- Season the chicken drumsticks and brown in the frying pan until golden brown on all sides.
- Place the browned chicken pieces in a large baking dish and set aside.
- Add another tablespoon of olive oil in the same frying pan and add in the onions and garlic and fry for 10 minutes.
- Add the lemon zest and juice, cumin and sherry to the onions and garlic and bring to the boil.
- Add in the almonds and the dates.
- Pour this sauce over the chicken drumsticks and cover with foil.
- Place in the preheated oven and cook for 50 minutes.

- Remove the foil and place back in the oven for another 15 minutes until all sticky and brown.
- Serve with a side dish of your choice.

ROSEMARY CHICKEN WITH A TOMATO SAUCE

YIELD: 4 SERVINGS

INGREDIENTS:
- 8 boneless chicken thighs
- 2 red onions, sliced fine
- 2 garlic cloves, sliced
- 1 anchovy fillets
- 1 can of chopped tomatoes
- 80ml of red wine
- 1 rosemary sprig, chopped
- 1 tablespoon of capers, drained
- 2 tablespoons of olive oil

DIRECTIONS:
- In a large frying pan on a medium to high heat, heat 1 tablespoon of the olive oil and brown the chicken pieces, add in the chopped rosemary and then set aside.
- In the same pan, add the remainder of the olive oil, add in the onion and garlic and gently fry for 5 minutes.
- Add in the anchovies and fry for 5 more minutes.
- Pour in the red wine, capers and the tomatoes and bring it to the boil.
- Return the chicken pieces to the pan and reduce the heat.
- Cover and gently simmer for 20 minutes.
- Serve with a crisp green salad and gluten free bread.

GLUTEN FREE MACARONI CHEESE

YIELD: 4 SERVINGS

INGREDIENTS:
- 1 packet of gluten free macaroni
- 5 tablespoons of butter
- 4 cups of skimmed milk
- 1/4 cup of cornstarch
- 3 1/2 cups of cheddar cheese, grated
- Salt and pepper for seasoning

DIRECTIONS:
- Preheat the oven to 180C degrees.
- Grease a casserole dish.
- Cook the gluten free macaroni according to the packet instructions, drain and set aside.
- In a medium sized saucepan on a medium heat, melt the butter and season with salt and pepper then set aside.
- In a separate mixing bowl, combine the cornstarch and milk and whisk until smooth.
- Stir the milk mixture into the butter mixture until well combined and smooth.
- Place the saucepan back onto the stove and cook on a medium heat until thickened stirring constantly.
- Stir in 3 cups of the grated cheddar cheese until the cheese has melted. Keep the remaining cheese for the topping.
- Combine the cheese sauce with the macaroni and pour into the prepared casserole dish.
- Top with the remaining cheddar cheese and season with salt and pepper.

- Bake in the preheated oven for 30 minutes.

CHICKEN AND LEEK PIE

YIELD: 4 SERVINGS

INGREDIENTS:

For the pie
- 180g of gluten free flour
- 90g of chilled butter, grated coarsely
- 60g of cheddar cheese, grated
- 1 tablespoon of wholegrain mustard

For the filling
- 500g of skinless, boneless chicken breasts, cut into chunks
- 30g of butter
- 2 tablespoons of olive oil
- 3 leeks, thickly sliced
- 300ml of chicken stock
- 1 tablespoon of gluten free flour
- 90g watercress, chopped
- 5 tablespoons of crème fraiche
- 2 tablespoons of milk

DIRECTIONS:
- Preheat the oven to 180C degrees.
- Mix the flour, butter and a pinch of salt into a bowl and then stir in the cheese. Blend in 2 tablespoons of cold water together with the mustard and combine. Form the mixture into a dough and chill for 30 minutes.
- In a frying pan on a medium to high heat, fry the chicken with the oil for 6 minutes until they are all golden.
- Add in the leeks and fry for 3 minutes until they are softened.

- Add in the stock and bring it to the boil, cover and reduce the heat and gently let it simmer for 15 minutes.
- Transfer the chicken and the leeks to a pie dish with a spoon, leaving the stock in the pan.
- Make a paste with the flour and one tablespoon of cold water.
- Add this to the stock in the pan and stir on a low heat until thickened.
- Take off the heat and stir in the watercress and the crème fraiche, season well..
- Pour the sauce over the chicken pieces and let it cool down.
- Roll out the chilled pastry until it will cover the pie dish. Carefully lay the rolled out pastry over your topping and trim around the rim.
- Make a small hole in the center of the pie and brush the pastry with the milk.
- Place in the preheated oven and cook for 30 minutes.

GLUTEN FREE PIZZA DOUGH

YIELD: 4 SERVINGS

INGREDIENTS:
- 1 1/2 cups of gluten free flour
- 2 teaspoons of xanthan gum
- 1 tablespoon of dry active yeast
- 1 envelope of plain gelatin
- 1/2 a teaspoon of honey
- 1 teaspoon of course salt
- 2 tablespoons of olive oil
- 2/3 warm water

DIRECTIONS:
- Preheat the oven to 200C degrees.
- Combine all of the ingredients into an electric mixer and mix on low until all the ingredients are well combined, scraping down the sides only once.
- With the mixer on high continue to mix for 3 minutes until it forms a dough.
- Dust a work surface with gluten free flour and knead the dough until smooth and no longer sticky. Press the dough into a pizza pan or baking sheet.
- Add any topping that you require.
- Bake for 15 to 20 minutes.

MEATBALL AND BUTTERBEAN STEW

YIELD: 3 SERVINGS

INGREDIENTS:
- 350g of lean pork mince
- 2 red onions, chopped
- 2 red peppers, chopped and deseeded
- 2 garlic cloves, crushed
- 1 tablespoon of paprika
- 2 tablespoons of olive oil
- 2 cans of chopped tomatoes
- 1 can of butter beans, drained
- 2 tablespoons of honey
- A bunch of fresh parsley, chopped

DIRECTIONS:
- Season the lean pork mince with salt and pepper and add in the paprika.
- Shape into small meatballs using your hands.
- In a large frying pan on a medium heat, add 1 tablespoon of olive oil and brown the meatballs until nice and golden. Set aside.
- In the same pan brown the onions and peppers until nice and soft then stir in the garlic.
- Add in the tomatoes, cover with a lid and let it simmer for 10 minutes.
- Stir in the beans and the honey and season if required.
- Simmer for an additional 10 minutes.
- Stir in the parsley.
- Serve warm.

MISO ROASTED AUBERGINE STEAKS WITH SWEET POTATO

YIELD: 2 SERVINGS

INGREDIENTS:
- 350g of sweet potatoes cut into wedges
- 2 aubergines
- 1 garlic clove, crushed
- 2 tablespoons of miso paste
- 1 teaspoon of freshly grated ginger
- 8 spring onions, sliced diagonally
- 2 tablespoons of olive oil
- 225ml boiling water
- A bunch of fresh parsley, chopped
- Salt and pepper to taste

DIRECTIONS:
- Preheat the oven to 180 C degrees.
- Peel the aubergines with a potato peeler and spread the miso paste on them with the back of a spoon.
- Place the aubergines in a baking tray with the sweet potato wedges.
- Pour in the boiling water and then add in the garlic and ginger. Sprinkle with salt and pepper and then place in the preheated oven.
- Bake for 35 minutes, then add an additional 125ml of boiling water and place back in for another 20 minutes.
- Take out and add in the spring onions and roast for an additional 10 minutes.
- Sprinkle with parsley and serve warm.

WARM QUINOA SALAD WITH HALLOUMI

YIELD: 3 SERVINGS

INGREDIENTS:
- 200g quinoa
- 1 red onion, sliced
- 1 roasted red pepper, sliced
- 500ml of vegetable stock
- Juice and Zest of 1 lemon
- 4 tablespoons of olive oil
- A pinch of sugar
- 250g of halloumi cheese, cut into 6 slices
- A handful of freshly cut parsley
- Salt and Pepper to taste

DIRECTIONS:
- In a saucepan on a medium to high heat add the olive oil.
- Cook the onion and the roasted pepper for a few minutes then add in the quinoa and cook for 4 minutes.
- Add the stock and reduce the heat, let it simmer gently for 15 minutes or until soft.
- Stir in half of the parsley.
- Preheat the grill
- In a separate bowl, combine the lemon zest and the juice along with the olive oil and the remaining parsley.
- Grill the halloumi on both sides until golden and crisp.
- Serve the salad with the grilled halloumi and pour the dressing over.

ROSEMARY LAMB CHOPS WITH ROASTED POTATOES

YIELD: 4 SERVINGS

INGREDIENTS:
- 10 lamb chops
- 1kg of potatoes, peeled and cut into wedges
- 3 rosemary sprigs
- 1 packet of cherry tomatoes
- 1 tablespoon of balsamic vinegar
- 4 tablespoons of olive oil
- 4 garlic cloves, left whole
- Salt and Pepper to taste

DIRECTIONS:
- Preheat the oven to 200C degrees.
- In a medium sized pan on medium to high heat, heat half of the oil and brown the lamb chops for 3 minutes on each side.
- Take out the pan and place in a roasting pan.
- Add the rest of the oil to the frying pan and add in the potatoes, fry them for 5 minutes.
- Add the rosemary and garlic to the potatoes and fry for 5 minutes.
- Season with salt and Pepper.
- Add the potatoes to the lamb shops.
- Roast in the oven for 20 minutes.
- Take out and add in the cherry tomatoes and balsamic vinegar.
- Place back in the oven for a further 10 minutes.
- Serve

10 Delicious Gluten Free Dessert Recipes

CHOCOLATE POTS

YIELD: 8 SERVINGS

INGREDIENTS:
- 2/3 cups of granulated sugar
- 2 tablespoons of corn starch
- 1/2 a teaspoon of kosher salt
- 3 cups of skim milk
- 4 egg yolks
- 1 teaspoon of vanilla essence
- 6 ounces of bittersweet chocolate, chopped
- 1 teaspoon of cocoa powder

DIRECTIONS:
- In a saucepan, on a medium heat, mix together the sugar, salt and corn starch.
- Add in 1/3 cup of the milk and stir until you get a nice paste.
- Whisk in the remaining milk and the egg yolks.
- Cook the mixture on a low heat, make sure to stir constantly with a wooden spoon until it is thick, this should take around 15 minutes, do not allow the mixture to boil.
- Remove from the heat.
- Add in the chopped chocolate and the vanilla essence and mix until the chocolate has melted.
- Pour into 8 ramekins and refrigerate for up to 3 hours.
- Sprinkle with cocoa powder just before serving.

POACHED PEARS

YIELD: 4 SERVINGS

INGREDIENTS:
- 1 1/4 cups of red wine
- 1 lemon
- 1 orange, quartered
- 3/4 cup of sugar
- 2 vanilla beans split
- 1 cinnamon stick
- 4 cloves
- 4 ripe pears, peeled

DIRECTIONS:
- In a saucepan, not on any heat, combine the juice from the lemon and the orange, wine, vanilla, sugar, cinnamon stick and the cloves.
- Add the pears to the saucepan with the liquid in it.
- Place on a medium heat and bring to the boil.
- Reduce the heat and let it simmer, uncovered, making sure to turn the pears occasionally.
- They should be soft and ready after about 25 minutes.
- Transfer the pears to individual plates.
- Remove the orange quarters and spices and discard.
- Place the remaining liquid back on to the stove and cook gently for around 15 minutes until you have a nice and thick syrupy mixture.
- Spoon the syrupy sauce over the pears and serve.

MAPLE AND WALNUT BAKED APPLES

YIELD: 4 SERVINGS

INGREDIENTS:
- 5 large apples
- 3/4 cup of maple syrup
- 1/4 cup of walnuts, chopped
- 1/3 cup of raisins
- 3 tablespoon of butter, chopped

DIRECTIONS:
- Preheat the oven to 180C degrees.
- Remove the cores from the apples and cut about a 1/2 inch slice from the bottom of each apple so that they can sit flat in an ovenproof baking dish.
- Pour the maple syrup over the apples.
- Combine the raisins and walnuts together and then put them in the apples cavities.
- Place a dot of butter on each apple.
- Bake in the oven for 40 minutes.
- Place the apples onto individual serving plates.
- Pour the remaining juices from the baked apples into a pot.
- Boil the liquid on a medium heat until the sauce thickens.
- Spoon the sauce over the warm apples.
- Serve with ice-cream.

PEACH AND RASPBERRY PARFAIT

YIELD: 4 SERVINGS

INGREDIENTS:
- 3 peaches, cut into pieces
- 2 cups of raspberries
- 2 tablespoons of sugar
- 2 tablespoons of lemon juice
- Ice cream to serve

DIRECTIONS:
- In a large mixing bowl, combine together the raspberries, peaches, sugar and the lemon juice.
- Let this sit for 20 minutes, stirring once during this time.
- Scoop ice cream into 4 individual serving bowls.
- Top with the fruit mixture.

RASPBERRY FOOL

YIELD: 4 SERVINGS

INGREDIENTS:
- 2 cups of raspberries
- 1/2 a cup of sugar
- 2 cups of whipped cream

DIRECTIONS:
- Mash the raspberries in a bowl and add in the sugar and combine together gently.
- Whip the cream to stiff peaks and fold into the raspberry mixture
- Spoon into individual glasses and serve.

EASY CHOCOLATE RICOTTA MOUSSE

YIELD: 4 SERVINGS

INGREDIENTS:
- 2 cups of ricotta cheese
- 3 tablespoons of icing sugar
- 5 ounces of chocolate, melted
- 1 ounce of chocolate, shaved for the topping

DIRECTIONS:
- Blend the ricotta cheese and melted chocolate in a food processor until smooth.
- Divide the mixture between bowls.
- Top with the shaved chocolate pieces.
- Refrigerate until ready to serve.

CARAMELIZED PINEAPPLE WITH A COCONUT SORBERT

YIELD: 4 SERVINGS

INGREDIENTS:
- 2 tablespoons of butter
- 1/4 cup of brown sugar
- 1 pineapple, cored and cut into wedges
- 1 pint of coconut sorbet

DIRECTIONS:
- Melt the butter in a pan over a medium heat, add in the sugar and cook for 2 minutes.
- Add in the pineapple wedges and cook until the pineapple is tender.
- Place the pineapple into individual bowls and serve with the remaining sauce and the coconut sorbet.

BUTTERMILK PUDDING

YIELD: 6 SERVINGS

INGREDIENTS:
- 1 envelope of unflavored gelatin
- 1 cup of heavy cream
- 2/3 cup of sugar
- 2 cups of buttermilk
- 1 1/2 teaspoons of vanilla essence
- Canola oil for the ramekins

DIRECTIONS:
- In a small mixing bowl, combine the gelatin with 1/4 cups of water and let it stand for 4 minutes.
- In a medium sized saucepan, combine the sugar with half of the cream.
- Cook on a low heat until the sugar has dissolved.
- Remove from the heat and whisk in the gelatin.
- In a large mixing bowl, combine the vanilla essence, remaining cream and the buttermilk.
- Stir the buttermilk mixture into the warm cream mixture.
- Get your 6 ramekins and slightly grease them with the canola oil.
- Divide your buttermilk mixture between the ramekins and refrigerate for 3 hours or overnight.

RASPBERRY SORBET WITH MERINGUES

YIELD: 8 SERVINGS

INGREDIENTS:
- 1 cup of whipped cream
- 2 tablespoons of icing sugar
- 16 small meringues
- 2 pints of raspberry sorbet

DIRECTIONS:
- In a mixing bowl, whip the cream and sugar together until soft peaks form.
- Ina separate mixing bowl, break the meringues gently into small pieces.
- In individual serving dishes, scoop the raspberry sorbet into each bowl.
- Spoon the whipped cream over the raspberry sorbet.
- Sprinkle the crumbled meringue over the cream.
- Serve immediately.

MANGO GRATIN

YIELD: 2 SERVINGS

INGREDIENTS:
- 1 ripe mango
- Juice and Zest of 1 lime
- 1 cup of vanilla yoghurt
- 2 tablespoons of butter
- 2 tablespoons of brown sugar

DIRECTIONS:
- Slice the mango lengthways around the side of the pit and remove the skin.
- Cut the mango into bite-size pieces and divide between two bowls.
- Stir in the lemon zest.
- Top with the yoghurt.
- Sprinkle the brown sugar on top of the yoghurt and dot with a teaspoon of butter onto each dish.
- Place under a grill for 3 minutes or until the top has turned a nice golden brown color.

10 Delicious Gluten Free Side Dish/Appetizer Recipes

SPINACH AND ARTICHOKE DIP

YIELD: 3 CUPS

INGREDIENTS:
- 1 packet of cooked chopped spinach
- 1 can of artichoke hearts, drained and chopped
- 1 cup of mayonnaise
- 1 cup of Parmesan cheese, grated
- 2 cups of Monterey Jack Cheese
- Salt and Pepper to taste

DIRECTIONS:
- Preheat the oven to 180C degrees.
- In a mixing bowl, combine the spinach, artichoke hearts, Parmesan cheese, mayonnaise and 1 1/2 cups of the Monterey Cheese and mix well.
- Place this mixture into a prepared baking dish and then sprinkle with the remaining Monterey Cheese.
- Bake in the preheated oven until the cheese has melted.
- Let the dip cool down and then serve with gluten free crackers or gluten free bread.

CRISPY BAKED KALE CHIPS

YIELD: 6 SERVINGS

INGREDIENTS:
- 2 bunches of Kale
- 2 tablespoons of olive oil
- 2 teaspoons of kosher salt

DIRECTIONS:
- Preheat the oven to 180C degrees.
- Grease a baking tray for the Kale.
- Tear the Kale into bite size pieces.
- Drizzle the Kale with the olive oil and sprinkle with the kosher salt.
- Bake for 15 minutes, the Kale leaves should be golden brown and crispy.

HAM ROLL UPS

YIELD: 4 SERVINGS

INGREDIENTS:
- 6 slices of cooked ham
- 1 packet of cream cheese, softened
- 6 dill pickles

DIRECTIONS:
- On a flat plat, lay the ham slices down and pat dry.
- Spread the ham with cream cheese and place a pickle onto each slice.
- Roll the slices into cylinders around the pickles and secure with a toothpick.

ASPARAGUS WRAPPED IN PROSCIUTTO

YIELD: 10 APPERTIZERS

INGREDIENTS:
- 10 asparagus spears
- 10 slices of prosciutto
- 2 tablespoons of olive oil

DIRECTIONS:
- Preheat the oven to 200C degrees.
- Line a baking sheet with aluminum foil.
- Coat the foil with the olive oil.
- Wrap the prosciutto slice around the asparagus spear and place on the prepared baking sheet.
- Bake for 5 minutes then take out and shake the baking tray so that the spears roll over.
- Bake for another 5 minutes until the spears are soft and the prosciutto is crisp.
- Serve immediately.

BACON AND DATES APPETIZERS

YIELD: YIELD 6 SERVINGS

INGREDIENTS:
- 1 package of pitted dates
- 1 cup of almonds
- 1 pound of sliced bacon

DIRECTIONS:
- Preheat the grill.
- Slit the dates and place one almond inside of the sliced date.
- Wrap the dates with the bacon slices and use toothpicks to secure them together.
- Grill in the preheated oven for 10 minutes, the bacon should be brown and crisp.

STUFFED CELERY

YIELD: YIELD 16 SERVINGS

INGREDIENTS:
- 1 package of cream cheese, softened
- 2 tablespoons of sour cream
- 1/2 a cup of walnuts, chopped
- 20 green olives
- 1 bunch of celery, cut into small bite size pieces

DIRECTIONS:
- In a mixing bowl mix together the sour cream with the cream cheese and add in the walnuts and olives.
- Spoon this filling into the celery pieces.
- Serve.

BEETROOT HUMMUS

YIELD: YIELD 8 SERVINGS

INGREDIENTS:
- 1 can of chickpeas, drained
- 1 red onion, finely sliced
- 1 pound of beets
- 1/2 a cup of tahini
- 4 garlic cloves, crushed
- 1/2 a cup of lemon juice
- 1 tablespoon of ground cumin
- 1/4 of a cup of olive oil
- Salt and Pepper to taste

DIRECTIONS:
- In a large saucepan, over a medium heat, add the beetroot and cover with water and boil until tender, drain the beets and remove the skins then chop them up.
- Puree in a blender all the ingredients except the olive oil, until nice and smooth.
- Slowly drizzle the olive oil in to the beetroot mixture.
- Pour into a serving dish and serve.

ROASTED SWEET ONION DIP

YIELD: YIELD 8 SERVINGS

INGREDIENTS:
- 3 sweet onions, peeled and quartered
- 2 tablespoons of olive oil
- 2 teaspoons of salt
- 3 garlic cloves, crushed
- 1/2 a cup of sour cream
- 1/4 cup of chopped fresh parsley
- 2 tablespoons of lemon juice

DIRECTIONS:
- Preheat the oven to 180C degrees.
- Place the onion into a mixing bowl and drizzle with the oil.
- Sprinkle the onions with 1 teaspoon of salt and toss to coat.
- Place the onion and garlic on a baking sheet.
- Bake for 1 hour in the preheated oven.
- Combine the garlic, onions, 1 teaspoon of salt, sour cream, lemon juice and parsley in a large bowl and mix together.
- Cover and chill for 1 hour before serving.

ROSEMARY, FENNEL AND CITRUS OLIVES

YIELD: YIELD 5 CUPS

INGREDIENTS:
- 4 cups of assorted olives
- 2 cups of olive oil
- 1 cup of fennel, chopped
- 2 teaspoons of fresh parsley, chopped
- 2 teaspoons of fresh rosemary, chopped
- 1 teaspoon of grated lemon rind
- 1 teaspoon of crushed red pepper
- 2 garlic cloves, crushed

DIRECTIONS:
- In a large mixing bowl, combine all of the above ingredients.
- Stir well to combine them all.
- Cover and refrigerate for 48 hours to marinade.
- Serve at room temperature.

HONEY ROASTED FRUIT AND NUTS

YIELD: YIELD 8 SERVINGS

INGREDIENTS:
- 2 teaspoons of butter
- 1/4 cup of honey
- 1/2 a cup of almonds, slivered
- 1/2 a cup of hazelnuts, chopped
- 1/2 a cup of pecans, chopped
- 1/4 cup of sunflower seed kernels
- 1 teaspoon of ground cardamom
- 1 teaspoon of ground cinnamon
- A dash of ground cloves
- 1 cup of raisons
- 1/4 teaspoon of salt
- Cooking spray

DIRECTIONS:
- Line a baking tray with parchment paper and coat with cooking spray.
- In a large nonstick pan over a medium to high heat, melt the butter and then stir in the honey and cook for 2 minutes.
- Add in all the remaining ingredients, except the raisons, and cook on a medium heat until all the nuts are coated and golden brown.
- Stir in the raisons.
- Spread onto the prepared baking tray and let them cool completely.
- Serve in a large bowl when cool.

Conclusion

Before I delve into the Conclusion I need to highlight an extremely important point. I'm doing this right here at the end of the book with the intention to leave it firmly and freshly in your mind. It is not okay to 'kind of' cut out Gluten, it must be 100% erased from your diet. Any small amount you consume will set off your Immune System's reaction again and you will be back at square one. Make the commitment to your health and go 100%!

A gluten-free diet will have definite changes from the diet you are accustomed to eating. That doesn't mean that you can't still have tasty foods that you enjoy.

Read the labels of foods you are purchasing, to ensure that they are gluten-free. Be careful not to fall for other phrasing like "wheat-free". If you have any questions, call the manufacturer. Their number will be on the packaging.

Plan meals ahead of time, and keep healthy, gluten-free foods in your refrigerator, or prepare meals and put them in your freezer. This way you will always have the makings for a good meal at home, even if you have to work late.

Stay positive about the changes you are making. If your food choices seem limited, remember how much better you feel when you eat foods that do not contain gluten.

Join others in your community and online who are also on gluten-free diets. You will get all kinds of cooking and baking ideas, and places where the foods you want are easily found. When you learn how many people who are going gluten free, like you are, it will make you feel less isolated and part of a group.

I hope I have convinced you to act. Please give a Gluten-Free diet a try and you will see the differences. Thank you for reading my book.

Free Ebook Offer
The Ultimate Guide To Vitamins

I'm very excited to be able to make this offer to you. This is a wonderful 10k word ebook that has been made available to you through my publisher, Valerian Press. As a health conscious person you should be well aware of the uses and health benefits of each of the vitamins that should make up our diet. This book gives you an easy to understand, scientific explanation of the vitamin followed by the recommended daily dosage. It then highlights all the important health benefits of each vitamin. A list of the best sources of each vitamin is provided and you are also given some actionable next steps for each vitamin to make sure you are utilizing the information!

As well as receiving the free ebooks you will also be sent a weekly stream of free ebooks, again from my publishing company Valerian Press. You can expect to receive at least a new, free ebook each and every week. Sometimes you might receive a massive 10 free books in a week!

All you need to do is simply type this link into your browser: http://bit.ly/18hmup4

Printed in Great Britain
by Amazon